CREEPY, KOOKY SCIENCE

Monstrous Medicine

Hannah Isbell

Enslow Publishing
101 W. 23rd Street
Suite 240
New York, NY 10011
USA
enslow.com

Published in 2020 by Enslow Publishing, LLC
101 W. 23rd Street, Suite 240, New York, NY 10011

Library of Congress Cataloging-in-Publication Data

Names: Isbell, Hannah, author.
Title: Monstrous medicine / Hannah Isbell.
Description: New York : Enslow Publishing, 2020. | Series: Creepy, kooky science | Audience: Grades 5 to 8. | Includes bibliographical references and index.
Identifiers: LCCN 2019009513| ISBN 9781978513785 (library bound) | ISBN 9781978513778 (pbk.)
Subjects: LCSH: Medicine—History—Juvenile literature. | Medicine—Miscellanea—Juvenile literature.
Classification: LCC R130.5 .I83 2020 | DDC 610.9—dc23
LC record available at https://lccn.loc.gov/2019009513

Printed in the United States of America

To Our Readers: We have done our best to make sure all websites in this book were active and appropriate when we went to press. However, the author and the publisher have no control over and assume no liability for the material available on those websites or on any websites they may link to. Any comments or suggestions can be sent by email to customerservice@enslow.com.

Photo Credits: Monstrous Medicine – Photo research by Bruce Donnola

Cover, p. 1 Gabdrakipova Dilyara/Shutterstock.com; pp. 6, 19 Science & Society Picture Library/Getty Images; p. 10 Peter Hermes Furian/Shutterstock.com; p. 11 Historical Picture Archive/Corbis Historical/Getty Images; p. 12 China Photos/Getty Images; p. 16 Leemage/Universal Images Group/Getty Images; p. 17 © AP Images; p. 23 Sergei Primakov/Shutterstock.com; p. 25 John Giles/PA Images/Getty Images; p. 26 Tacio Philip Sansonovski/Shutterstock.com; p. 31 Stock Montage/Archive Photos/Getty Images; p. 33 Alila Medical Media/Shutterstock.com; p. 35 BSIP SA/Alamy Stock Photo; p. 37 Kateryna Kon/Shutterstock.com; p. 39 Design_Cells/Shutterstock.com

Contents

Introduction

For most of human history, the majority of people led very short lives. Without vaccines to prevent common diseases, most children died before they turned five years old. Without knowledge of germs and how they spread, infection and illness were a part of everyday life.

Pus, boils, rotting teeth, itchy rashes, and diarrhea were common. So were terrible injuries and wounds. Plagues could wipe out entire towns and cities. And without a good understanding of how the human body works, doctors and healers weren't very successful at treating their patients. People were lucky to live into their forties! But about two hundred and fifty years ago, something changed: humans began to use modern medicine.

Before modern medicine, most people believed illness was caused by evil spirits, angry gods, or bad energy. Different cultures and communities had different ideas about what caused diseases and how to treat them, but across cultures, religious figures like shamans and priests were the first doctors. They treated their sick and injured patients according to their religious beliefs. Prayers, exorcisms, rituals, and sacrifices were made to try to keep people and communities healthy.

Humans of the past also used what they could find in nature. Sometimes, they were very successful. More than two thousand years ago, ancient Sumerians, Egyptians, and indigenous Americans all used willow plants to treat pain and fevers. Now the same willow is used to make aspirin! Archaeologists have even discovered evidence of successful surgery done over ten thousand years ago! Prehistoric skulls have been found with holes drilled into them. This was a medical treatment called trepanning. Trepanning was sometimes done to treat a person who had mental illness because people believed spirits trapped in the head were causing the disease.[1] This, of course, was not the case.

Though not helpful for mental illness, trepanning was used in successful emergency surgery. In prehistoric and ancient times, head wounds from spears, slingshots, and other hard items were common. Just as a bruise can form after a person has taken a hard hit, bleeding can also happen inside the skull. This bleeding can press on the brain, which is dangerous and even deadly. Prehistoric and ancient surgeons would drill holes into the skull to relieve the pressure. Modern surgeons relieve pressure from bleeding inside the skull in a similar way.

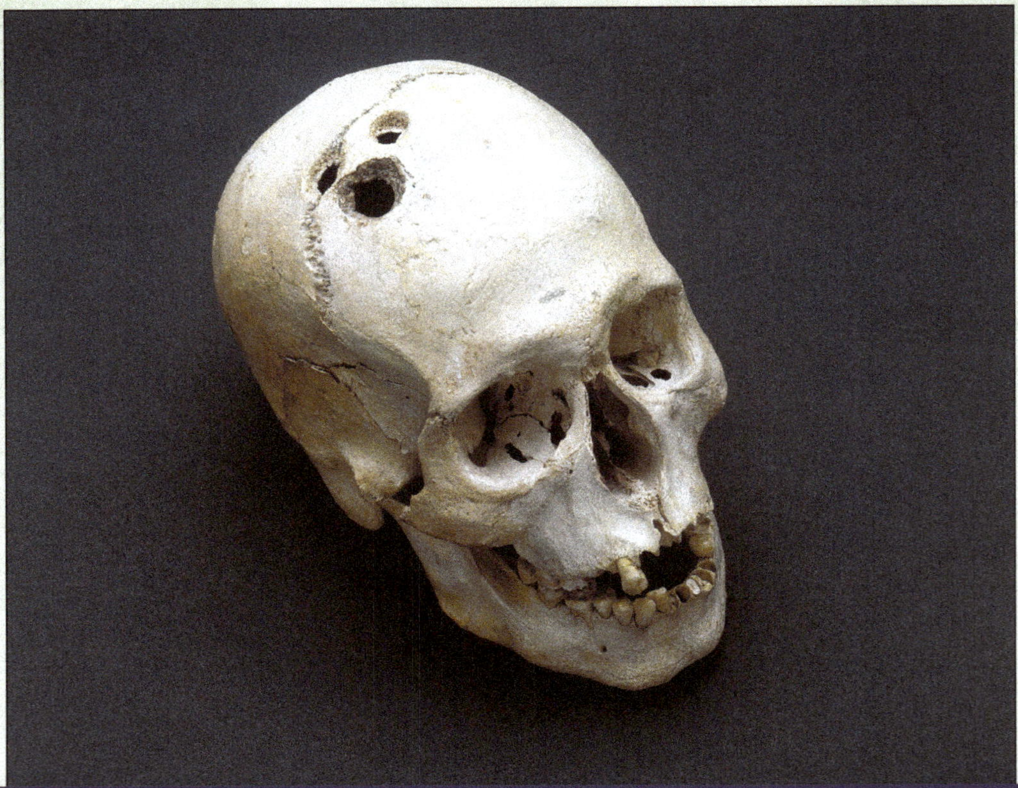

A Bronze Age skull bears several holes from trepanning. The skull, which is about four thousand years old, was found in the West Bank in Israel. The bone shows evidence of healing, which means this person survived the procedure.

But sometimes, people of the past weren't so successful. Terrible potions made of toxic mercury, ointments made of animal dung, radioactive salves, and brews made of ground-up Egyptian mummies were all used as medicine! Ancient humans weren't stupid, but they lacked one very important tool that people have today: the scientific method. This is the process used to understand nature by making observations, taking measurements, and conducting experiments.

Science has led to the discovery that bacteria, viruses, toxins, and genetic problems are what make people sick. Doctors and scientists have technology that allows them to see deep inside bodies, into cells, and into the genes that make individuals who they are—and that often determines whether they are sick or healthy.

In the past hundred years, modern medicine has doubled the average lifespan to about eighty. Many people in developed countries today may even live past one hundred! However, modern medicine has seen many missteps, bizarre ideas, and terrifying treatments, too. Upon first glance, some of the most cutting-edge treatments of today can appear as strange and monstrous as the practices of the past.

What if a doctor wanted to inject a patient with bee venom? Or attached part of a pig's heart to a person's heart? Or implanted a mind-reading microchip in someone's brain? Or asked a patient to swallow a pill made of someone else's poop? These are all real, successful, modern medical treatments! How did doctors get here, and what does the future of medicine hold?

CHAPTER 1

Horrible History

No one knows exactly when humans started using medicine, but it was many thousands of years ago. Evidence of early medicine can be seen in bones from the Stone Age. The first known dental work dates back nine thousand years! Ancient treatments can be found written in books, on scrolls, and carved into stone tablets. All across the ancient world—from India, China, and Mesopotamia, to Egypt, Greece, and the Americas—people were making important discoveries, and terrible mistakes, in medicine.

Some of the things that people tried may seem silly or even stupid today. However, making mistakes and trying new things is how people learn and make progress. The strange ideas of the past led to some curious and monstrous medicine, but those same strange ideas led to great discoveries, too.

Spirits, Humors, and Unearthly Energies

Modern doctors know that viruses, bacteria, and other toxins in the environment cause disease. Disease can also be caused by problems in people's genes. Sometimes it is both genes and the environment coming together that cause illnesses.

However, before the invention of the microscope, people didn't know that germs existed or that bodies were made up of cells. They didn't have a good understanding of anatomy or the way the body is put together and how it works.

Ancient people got many things wrong. For example, the ancient Egyptians thought the brain's only job was keeping the body cool. They thought so little of the brain that when they mummified bodies, they took the brain out and threw it away! The ancient Greeks thought it was the heart, not the brain, that created thoughts and feelings.

People of the past got some things right, though. They *did* know that some illnesses could run in families, but they didn't understand why or how. They also knew that diseases could be contagious, meaning they could spread from one person to another. Thousands of years ago, the Mesopotamian people even took steps to prevent the spread of disease. An example of this is

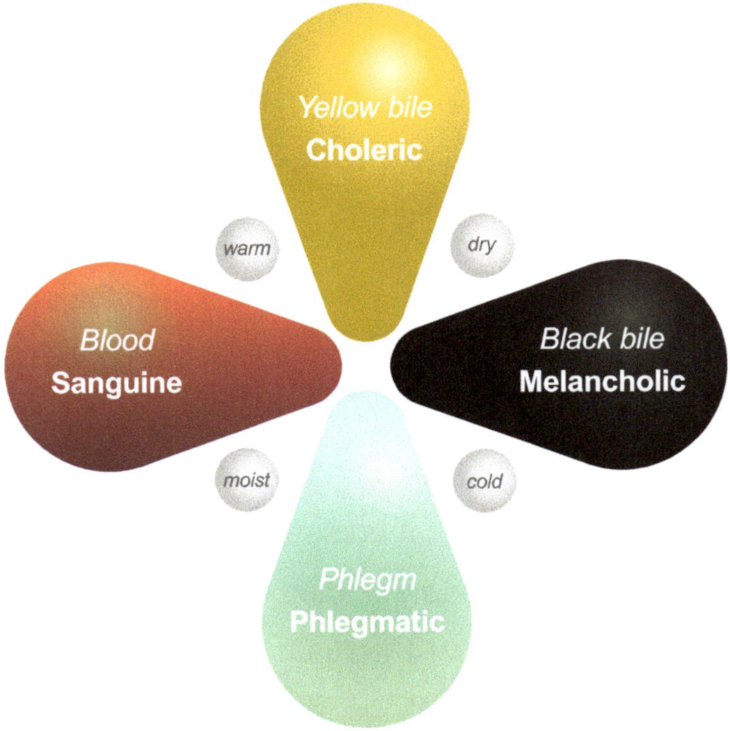

The humors were bodily fluids once thought to work together to make people healthy. Humors were classified in opposites: warm or cold, and dry or moist. The opposites described the emotional traits of the humors, too. Sanguine means positive or happy, while melancholic means gloomy and sad. Choleric means irritable, while phlegmatic means calm.

their use of quarantine, which is when sick people, or even entire towns or cities, are separated from healthy people.

Around the world, however, people believed things such as bad spirits, gods, and unbalanced energy caused disease. The ancient Mesopotamians thought their gods were responsible for mental illness. Ancient Americans also believed illness was caused by spirits. Many cultures had similar beliefs. But the most important ideas in pre-scientific medicine were about the balance of energies and humors.[1]

Weird and Wild Remedies

Humorism sounds funny, but "humor" has another meaning. For more than a thousand years, it was believed that good health relied on balancing four bodily fluids, called humors. The four humors were black bile, yellow bile, phlegm, and blood. From ancient Greece through the Middle Ages, doctors used humorism to understand disease and treat patients. This led to some pretty wild remedies!

Bloodletting is probably one of the most famous treatments based in humorism. It was one of the most common medical treatments for nearly two thousand years. Doctors stopped regularly practicing bloodletting only a little more than two hundred years ago. If a doctor thought too much blood caused a patient's illness, the doctor would apply blood-sucking leeches or even cut open a patient's arm to let some of the blood out. Doctors would use

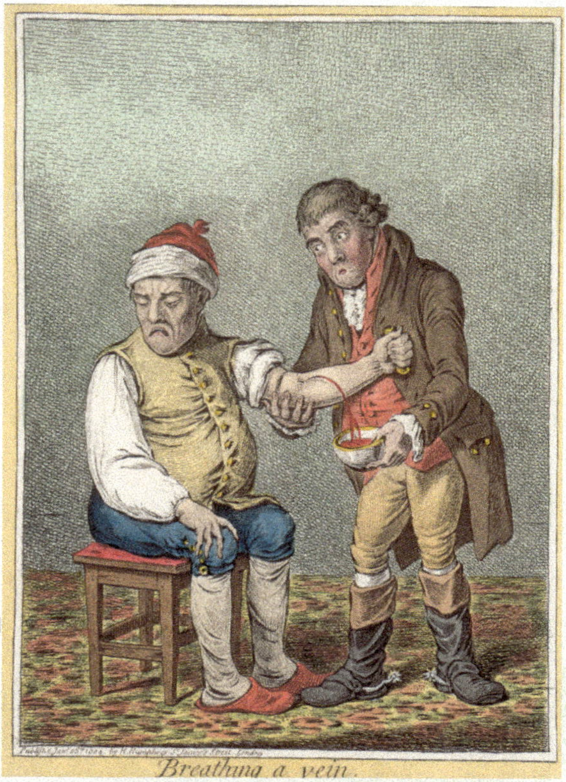

This work by British artist James Gillray (1756–1815) is titled *Breathing a Vein* (1804). It shows a doctor using bloodletting to treat a patient. Having pierced a vein, the doctor collects the blood in a bowl.

bloodletting to treat anything from heart disease to a bad cough!

Cupping was another way doctors tried to balance humors. They believed that suction, the same force that lets one suck a drink through a straw, could pull out toxins they thought were causing an imbalance of the humors. Placing hot cups on patients' backs and backsides would create the suction. The terrible bruises they caused were believed to be evidence of the toxins coming out of the body.[2] In an even grosser twist, some people would pierce the skin before placing the cup, in a practice called *hijama*,

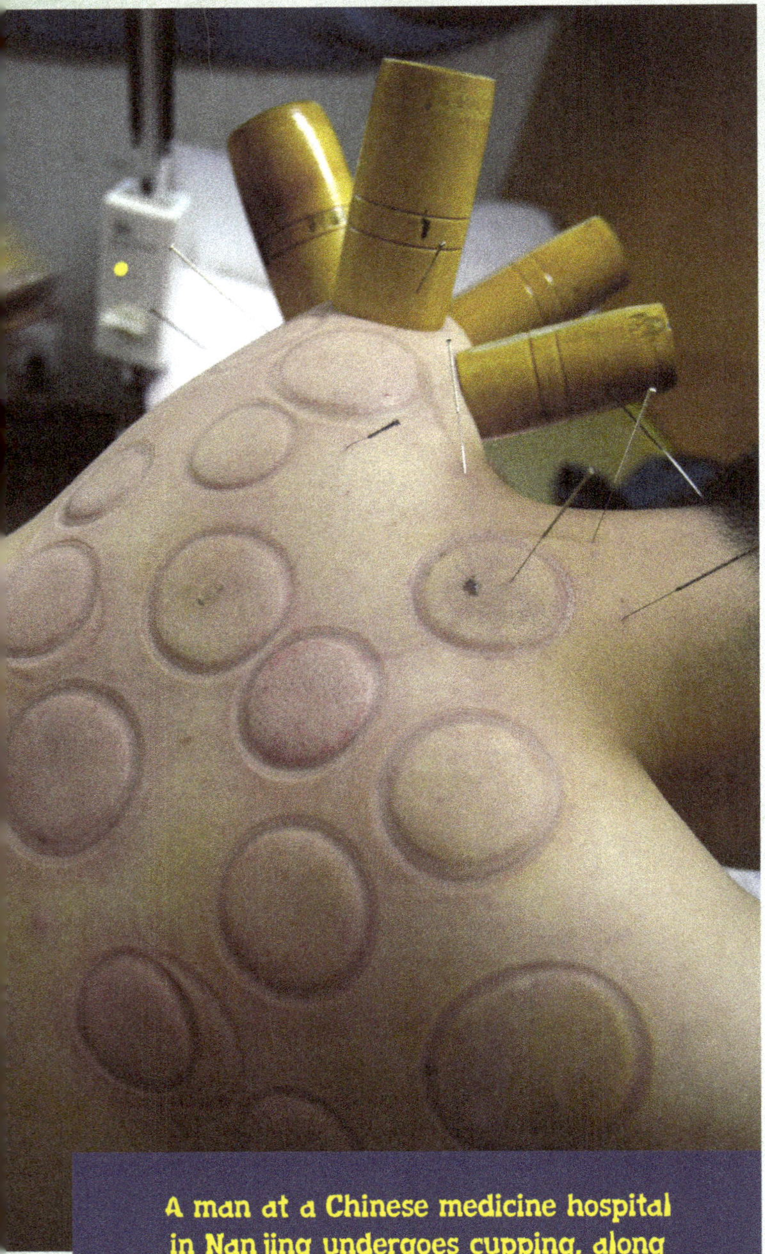

A man at a Chinese medicine hospital in Nanjing undergoes cupping, along with acupuncture. People use cupping to treat everything from pain to infection, but science doesn't support cupping as either safe or effective.

or wet cupping. Cutting the skin first allows the suction to pull the blood out and into the cup, which is another way of bleeding a patient.[3]

Cupping has been used for three thousand years, and people still try cupping today. There is no evidence that it works, though, and in rare cases, it can cause terrible and even deadly problems such as blood clots and rotting ulcers!

Medical Principles

Ancient Indians were the first to use some of the most basic and important ideas in medicine. They came up with the idea of diagnosis, or studying symptoms to identify diseases. They also came up with the idea of prognosis, an educated guess about how the disease or injury might progress.

Ancient Indians were also the first to use medical ethics. Medical ethics are rules that ensure patients are treated well and with respect. Other cultures adopted similar ideas. The Hippocratic Oath, an oath to use good ethics, was written about five thousand years ago in ancient Greece. A form of the oath, in which doctors vow to help their patients and do no harm, is still taken today.

Strange Successes

At the same time that people had some strange ideas about medicine, they also came up with ideas and practices doctors still use today. There is evidence from around the world of people using the tools and resources they had in clever and successful ways.

Some of the first successes in medicine were probably treatments for injuries. Ancient humans led very active and dangerous lives. Hunting and gathering in the wild could lead to trips and falls and encounters with dangerous wild animals. Fighting with other people could lead to broken bones, cuts, and gashes.

Ancient Asian tribes were the first to cauterize. They would mix sulfur and other minerals, put the mixture on a wound, and set it on fire. Cauterizing stops wounds from bleeding and removes dead flesh. Cauterizing is still an important way of treating wounds today.

Ancient Americans used quills from feathers to drain infections. They also came up with a gross but brilliant way to stitch up wounds using biting insects! They would hold an ant against a wound so that it would bite the edges. Then they would twist the ant's body off, leaving the head and pincers as a stitch. It was effective, though it must have been extremely painful!

The history of medicine is a hodgepodge of wacky ideas and brilliant breakthroughs. When people started using science in medicine, they were able to begin sorting out what really worked from what was just really weird. And sometimes, real remedies seem just as strange as the wildest ideas from history.

CHAPTER 2

Gross Elixirs and Ointments

Before scientific medicine, people created many strange creams, ointments, potions, and pills. Herbalism, the use of plants as medicines, was important in all cultures around the world. Different parts of plants were put directly on the skin or on wounds, or made into drinks or pills. Many plants really can help with pain, fevers, swelling, and keeping wounds clean. Many modern medicines are made from those plants.

Some herbalism was not so successful. People believed, for example, that if a plant looked like a part of the human body, it could treat illness in that part of the body. This belief was called the doctrine of signatures. At best, this led to people taking useless potions and pills. At worst, it led to people using toxic plants as medicine and doing more harm than good.

People also used other things found in nature to make medicinal drinks and ointments, including some things that would sound downright disgusting to people today!

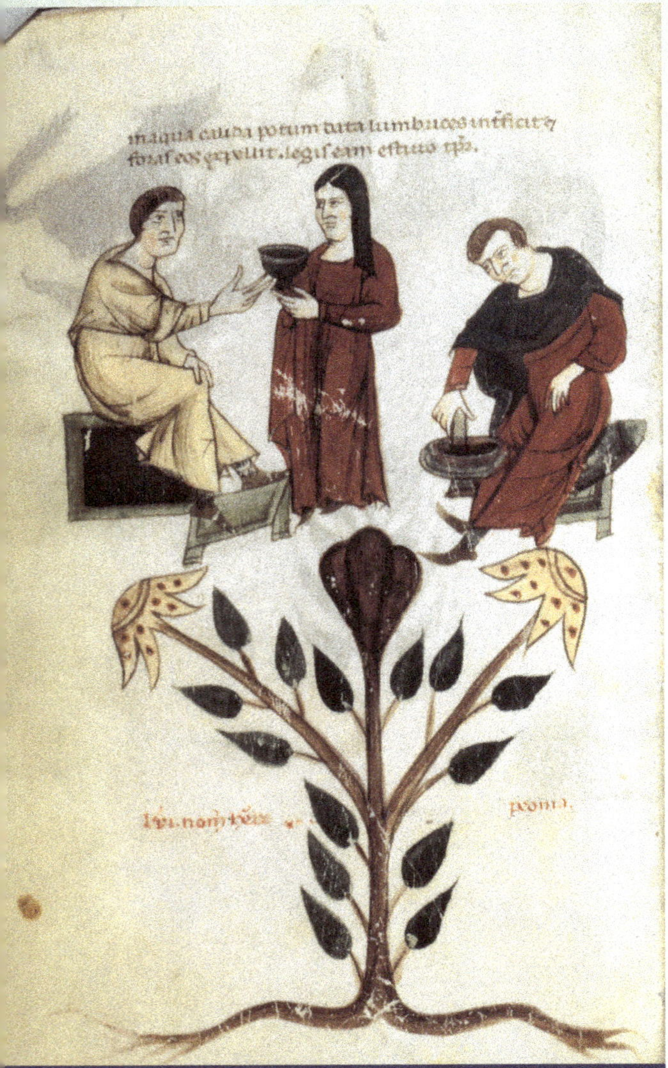

A document written in Latin shows an illustration of a peony plant and people using it to make a medicinal potion. Peonies were thought to help with arthritis, gout, and cramps.

Strange Salves

Early physicians made some great discoveries. In ancient Egypt, they knew that honey could keep a wound from becoming infected. Modern science has confirmed that honey really is antibacterial! But some of the treatments applied to wounds, rashes, and the skin of the sick were dirty, dangerous, and even deadly.

It's hard to imagine, but for a long time, one of the most common ointments used to treat wounds was made of … poop. Animal dung ointments were made from the feces of various animals, including goats, donkeys, dogs, and crocodiles. Even human dung was used as medicine. Just a few hundred years ago, a doctor in Europe might prescribe mashed baby dung for epilepsy or blow powdered people poop into ailing eyes.

A Hard Pill to Swallow

Even deadlier than dung was heavy metal medicine. Some metals are actually a natural part of the human body. Gold, copper, and iron are all normal things to find in people and are even important to health. But metals can be toxic if doses are too high, or if they are swallowed. Unfortunately, people of the past didn't know this. Elixirs made of toxic mercury and silver were common. These metals could cause terrible side effects such as brain damage and nerve damage. They could even cause death.

Silver Poisoning

One of the stranger side effects of heavy metal medicine comes with drinking silver. To this day, some people believe drinking silver can cure diseases, but there is no evidence that it works, and it is extremely dangerous. Drinking high doses of silver can actually turn a person's skin blue! Sadly, turning blue is just the start, because drinking silver can be deadly, too.

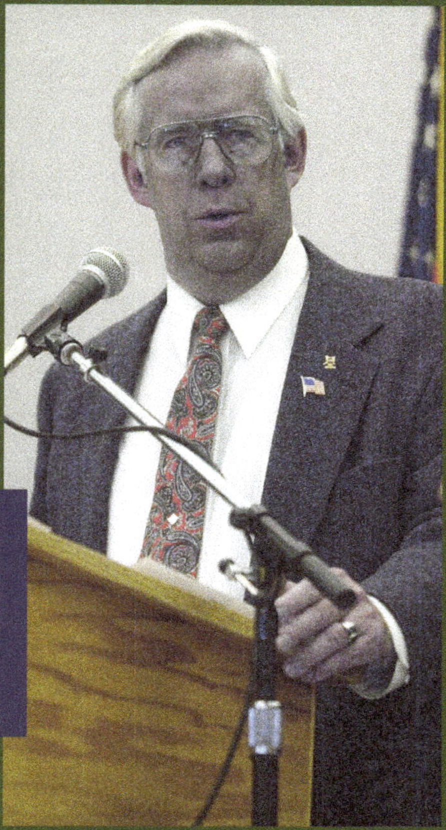

Stan Jones was a Libertarian candidate for the US Senate in 2002. His skin shows the blue tinge of colloidal silver. He began taking the silver over fears of an antibiotics shortage.

Though not as deadly as mercury or silver, another metal called antimony was used to treat tummy troubles for hundreds of years. It was made into a pill and swallowed. Antimony is a rare and expensive metal, though, so people wouldn't just throw something made of antimony away. After the pill passed through a person's system, they'd rummage through their dung to find it, so it could be used again. Antimony pills were passed down through families in this way for generations.[1]

Drinking the Dead

Possibly one of the most horrific medical practices of all time was corpse medicine. It may seem especially strange today, but for a long time, people believed the bodies of the dead had healing properties. Indeed, the reason ancient Egyptian mummies are rare today is because for hundreds of years people used to eat them!

Mummification is a way that bodies can be preserved after death. Mummified bodies don't decay, or rot normally. There may be a couple reasons that people came to believe mummies could heal. Some of the chemicals used by ancient Egyptians to mummify their dead could be antibacterial, lending a grain of truth to the idea that mummies could help with wounds.

People also didn't understand how natural mummification worked. When they found bodies preserved by freezing or in bogs, they thought that only a miracle could have kept the body from decaying. They hoped to treat their own health with that miraculous power.

Mummy powder was made by grinding up mummified bodies. It was brewed into drinks, eaten, and made into ointments to treat all sorts of illnesses.[2]

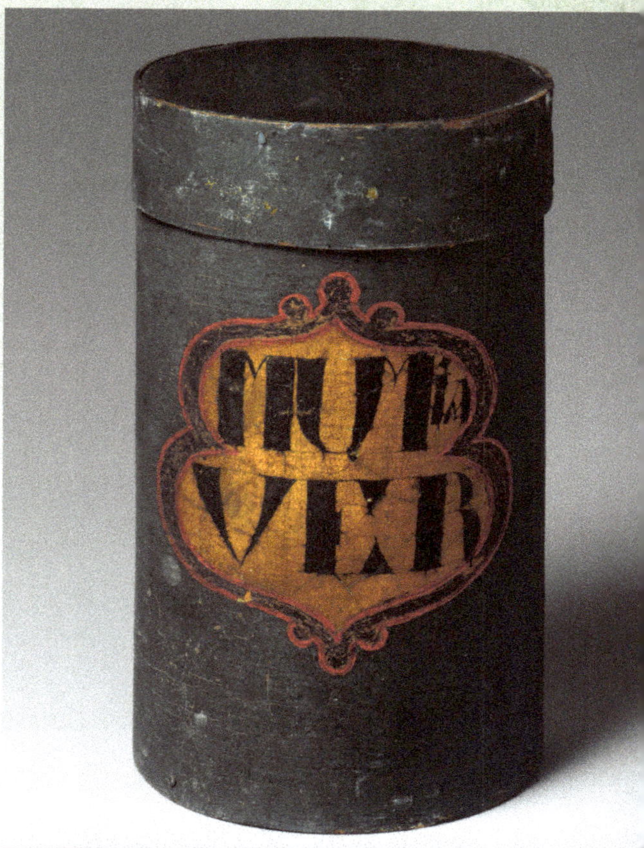

This wooden box, which once contained powdered mummy, is from Europe. It dates from about 1600 to 1800.

Homeopathy

Just a few hundred years ago, a doctor in eastern Europe created a new type of medicine, and it resulted in some interesting pills and potions. This pre-scientific medicine was called homeopathy, and the people who practiced it were called homeopaths.

Homeopathy is based on two ideas, and both of those are a bit backward. The first idea is that the cause of an illness is also the cure. For example, if a homeopath wanted to treat a bee allergy, then bee venom would be used in making a homeopathic remedy. The second idea was that mixing treatments with water, also called diluting, made them stronger. Homeopaths believed that the more something was diluted in water, the more powerful it became. This, of course, is the opposite of what really happens. Homeopaths actually diluted their medicines in so much water that there was usually none of the original medicine left.[3]

However, in a time when doctors were prescribing poisonous plants, toxic metals, animal poo powders, and mummy medicine, most patients were better off getting just plain water! This might be part of the reason some people still believe in homeopathy today, even though there is no evidence that it works.

Pus and Pox

One of the most famous cases of gross-but-good medicine was the discovery of the smallpox vaccine. Before the vaccine, smallpox was one of the deadliest diseases known to humanity. It caused high fever and pus-filled blisters all over the body. It spread very easily. About one in three people who caught smallpox died. Those who lived were left with terrible scars and sometimes blinded.

A vaccine is a way to protect a person from disease. When a person becomes ill, the body's defense, called the immune system, works to fight the disease. A vaccine works by exposing the body to a weak form of a disease-causing bacteria or virus. This allows the immune system to learn to fight the disease in a safer way. Once the immune system has learned to fight a disease, the vaccinated person can be exposed to it without becoming ill. This is called being immune.

Many people, over hundreds of years, contributed knowledge to the discovery of the smallpox vaccine. The first person to write about preventing smallpox was Wan Quan, a Chinese author writing in the sixteenth century. He described doctors taking scabs from people who had smallpox and making them into a powder. Then the doctors would blow the powder up the noses of new patients. These patients would get sick, but usually not as sick as if they'd caught smallpox in another way, and fewer of them died.

About two hundred years later in England, a doctor named Edward Jenner (1749–1823) made the first modern vaccine. He knew that people who caught a disease called cowpox were immune to smallpox. In the year 1796, he took pus from a woman suffering cowpox and injected it into a boy named James Phipps. James later proved to be immune to smallpox.

For two hundred years, the vaccine was used around the world. In one of the greatest feats of modern medicine, smallpox was wiped out in 1979. Because of the vaccine, no one in the world has been sick or died from smallpox in more than forty years.

Unfortunately, ever since the first vaccine, some people have been afraid of them. It is understandable because the idea of having a bacteria or virus injected on purpose is a little gross, strange, and even scary. However, vaccines are very safe. Modern medicine now has vaccines for many of the deadliest diseases a person can catch, and these vaccines have saved millions of lives!

CHAPTER 3

Leeches, Maggots, and Beneficial Beasts

Cowpox, as one might guess from the name, is a disease people caught when working with cows. Without cowpox, a smallpox vaccine may never have been discovered. Humans have used animals in medicine for thousands of years, from ancient animal sacrifices done to calm the angry spirits they believed caused illness to dung remedies of the Middle Ages. Animals are still used in medicine in modern times. Some of the most useful animals are also the most surprising.

Leeches

Leeches have been used in medicine for more than two thousand years. Leeches were once used in bloodletting, but when doctors learned that bloodletting wasn't helpful, the use of leeches became outdated. For more than a hundred years, leeches were thought of as a medical misstep, but modern medicine has found new uses for these bloodsuckers.

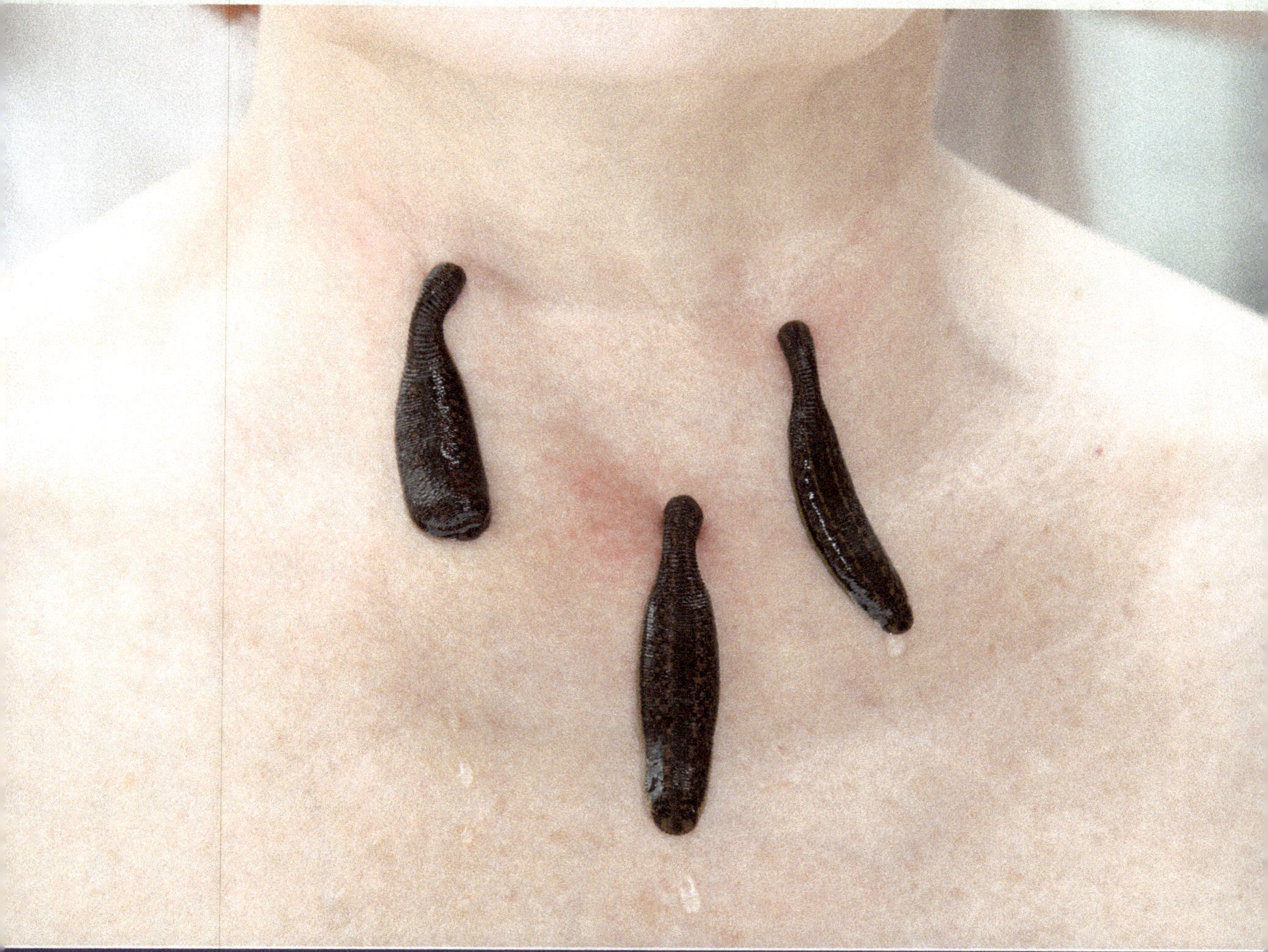

Leeches on a woman's neck may look gross, but they usually do not cause too much irritation and often can't be felt at all!

A leech feeds by sticking suckers on either end of its body into a human or animal. The leech's saliva has a painkiller in it. This helps keep the person or animal, called a host, from noticing the slimy creature attached to their body. The leech also injects a blood thinner into the host, letting it drink more from one spot. These are the weird features of leeches that make the creatures useful today.

Leeches work well in surgeries such as skin grafts and reattaching fingers and other body parts. The leech can be used as an artificial vein. It can keep blood flowing to the skin graft or the reattached body part so that the flesh doesn't die and the wound can heal.[1]

Maggots

Skin grafts are often used to treat burns and other large, open wounds by covering the wound and keeping out infection. Infection is one of the greatest risks of a burn or open wound. Another risk is necrosis.

Necrosis means death. If the flesh around a wound starts to die, it can keep the wound from healing. Because of this, doctors need to remove all the dead flesh from around a burn or wound. This can be difficult and messy. It can be hard to tell which flesh can be saved and what needs to go. This is where maggots come in.

Maggots, the larvae of flies, are usually found on the rotting corpses of animals, in dumpster bins, and anywhere else death and decay are around. So, a person might be surprised to find them in a hospital! What makes maggots so useful is that they eat dead flesh, and *only* dead flesh. Maggots can be poured on top

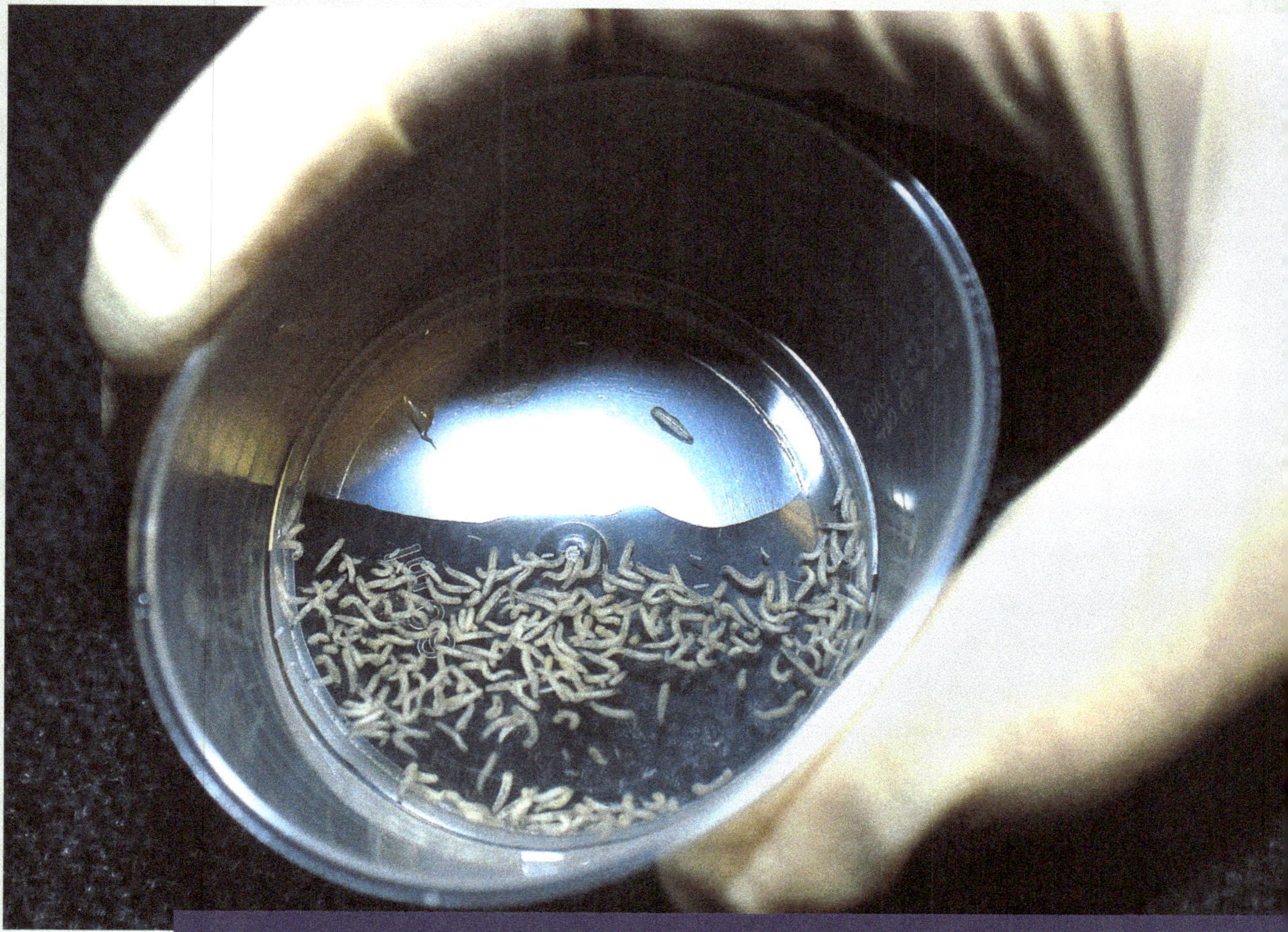

A researcher at the University of York holds a sample of maggots. The maggots are to be used in cleaning leg ulcers and may be cheaper and more effective than more common methods!

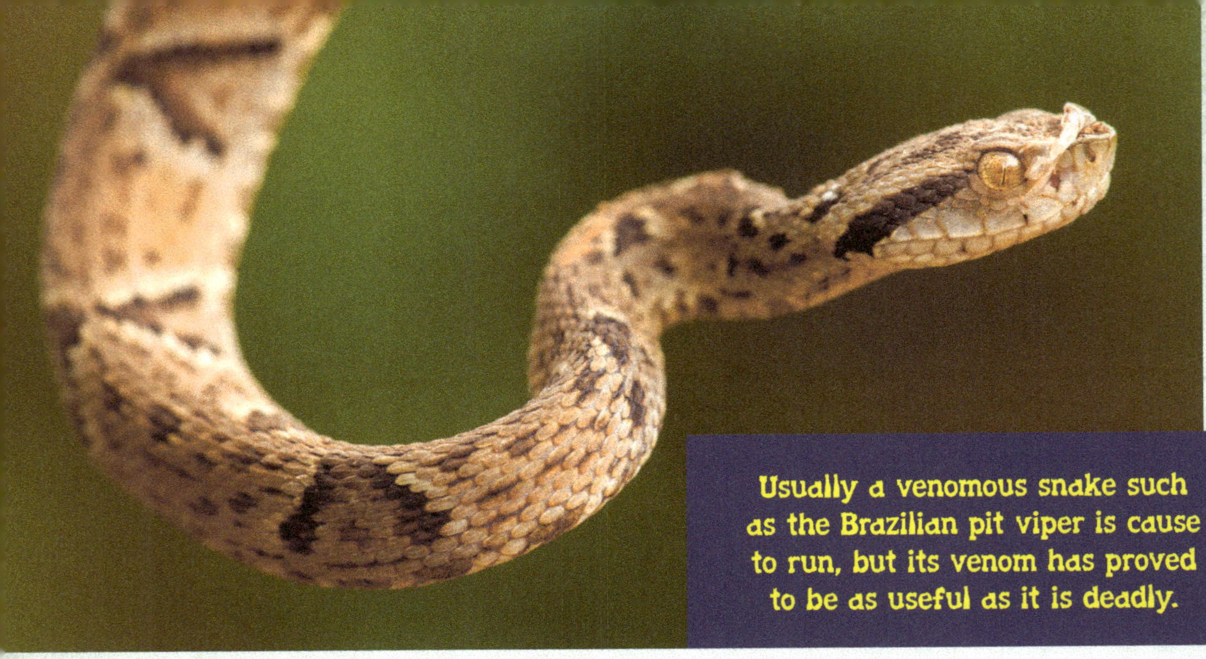

Usually a venomous snake such as the Brazilian pit viper is cause to run, but its venom has proved to be as useful as it is deadly.

of burns and other wounds and will clean away all the dead flesh. They will leave the living flesh alone so that it can begin to heal.

Virtuous Venom

Beestings and snakebites may hardly seem helpful, but in the past few decades, people have been finding surprising medical uses for venom. Venom is any toxic substance made by animals to defend themselves against other animals. It is often delivered through a bite or a sting. Many beasts, including insects, snails, lizards, frogs, and snakes, produce venom.

Just as humans turned to nature and found medicine in some plants, people are now finding medicine in some venom, too. But this doesn't mean anyone should let a snake bite them or a bee sting them!

Venom is made up of lots of stuff: proteins and other molecules that work in different ways. Scientists spend years carefully studying what about the venom can be helpful. They work hard to separate the helpful parts, separating the good from the bad. One toxin in the venom from the Brazilian pit viper lowers blood pressure, and low blood pressure can kill. Some people suffer from high blood pressure, though, and so a drug that lowers blood pressure can be useful. Scientists studied the viper venom and learned how to turn the dangerous substance into a helpful medicine.

Doctors can now treat pain with a medicine made from cone snail venom. They can treat diabetes with a medicine made from the venom of a lizard called a gila monster. And they can even use medicine made from rattlesnake venom to prevent heart attacks!

The creators of these medicines must not only be careful about isolating the helpful parts of the venom, but they must also be careful about the dose. Just like with medicines made from plants, sometimes something that is helpful in tiny amounts is dangerous or deadly in large amounts. Sometimes the difference between a medicinal dose and a deadly dose is tiny!

The Sad Story of the White Rhino

In Asia, many people believe the horn of the white rhinoceros can treat a host of different diseases and injuries. White rhinos are poached for their horns, which are sold for hundreds of thousands of dollars. The horns are powdered and made into pills, creams, and elixirs. There is no evidence white rhino horn can treat illness or injury, though.

White rhinos have been hunted almost to extinction. There are only a few thousand southern white rhinos in the wild. And sadly, there are only two northern white rhinos alive today.[2]

Snake Oil

Modern medicine has shown how ancient animal remedies can actually work, as well as finding new, amazing ways to use bugs and beasts. There have been medical missteps, such as using leeches to bleed patients, and medical marvels, such as using the same leeches to help blood reach a reattached finger. Some medical missteps, however, have done terrible harm to both humans and animals. Fake medicine is especially harmful.

Sometimes, fake medicine, which is also called snake oil or quackery, comes from people not understanding how diseases and bodies work. Just like people of the past got some things wrong, people today can get things wrong, too. Other times, it comes from people who want to fool others into buying fake medicine or treatments.

The term "snake oil" became popular in the nineteenth century. In China, people had long used the fat from the Chinese water snake to treat pain. However, in the nineteenth century, people in Europe and the Americas started to make fake snake oil treatments. They were usually useless combinations of oils and herbs and sold at very high prices. Snake oil salesmen claimed their oils could treat every disease! Today, "snake oil" is a term used to describe fake medicines and false claims. Many people have died because they used snake oil treatments instead of real medicine.

It is very important to remember that, while snake venom can really be turned into a useful drug, snake oil is something different, and the results of snake oil really can be monstrous.

CHAPTER 4

Barbary and Bedlam

Snake oil and quackery prey on people's lack of knowledge about the body and how it works. It took thousands of years of observation and two hundred years of modern medical science before experts had a good understanding of the body. Even now, there is much to be discovered. The human body is very complex, made up of cells, organs, and systems. Scientists are learning more about it every day.

Of all the organs and systems, the most complicated is the human brain. There are more neurons in the human brain than there are stars in the galaxy. It is the brain that allows humans to make sense of the world. It is the primary organ responsible for thoughts, emotions, and behavior. For these reasons, the medical missteps in mental health are among the most terrible, terrifying, and barbaric.

Bedlam

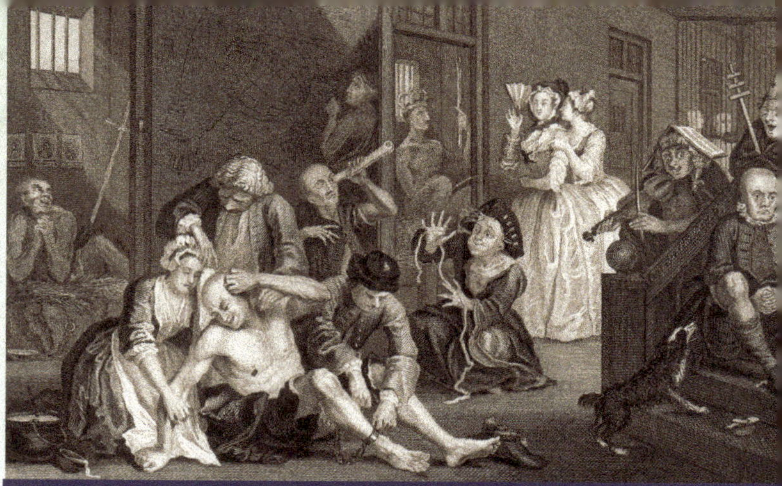

An engraving made from a painting by William Hogarth (1697-1764) shows a scene from Bethlem Royal Hospital in the 1730s. Some patients are shown to be suffering terribly, while others are made to perform for visitors.

Today the word "bedlam" means "wild confusion, or disaster." The word comes from the nickname for an early London mental hospital, Bethlem Royal Hospital, which was founded nearly eight hundred years ago. Given how people with mental illness were treated, it is no surprise the word has come to mean chaos.

In the past, mental illness was deeply misunderstood. Like physical illness, people often believed mental illness was caused by bad sprits or gods. Exorcisms were a common treatment.

For a long time, people even believed the moon caused mental illness. This is where the words "lunatic" and "lunacy" come from. Even today, many people believe there is a connection between the full moon and bad behavior, though there is no evidence that this is true.

In the past, patients in lunatic asylums were treated more like prisoners. They were kept away from others, often tied up, chained, or restrained in special garments called straitjackets.

They were forced to take ice baths, starved, and even beaten. People would pay to go and see them, like animals in a zoo.

In the eighteenth and nineteenth centuries, ideas about mental health started to change. People began to look at mental illness as a moral problem and thought it could be treated by teaching moral discipline and by working with the patient to change their beliefs. While this treatment didn't get everything right, it was much more humane and could even be helpful. Today, it is known that mental illness is not a moral issue, but talking about a patient's thoughts, feelings, and behaviors are often the foundations of modern, and effective, mental health treatment.

Lobotomies

In 1949, doctors began performing one of the most infamous treatments of the twentieth century, the lobotomy. A lobotomy is a surgery that cuts connections in the prefrontal cortex, which is the part of the brain that controls much of a person's thinking and behavior. While the procedure could be effective at controlling mental illness, it did so at the price of damaging the person's intellect and changing their personality.

Lobotomies became very popular in the mid-twentieth century, with more than twenty thousand being done in the United States alone. They were used to treat a wide range of mental illnesses, from depression to psychosis.

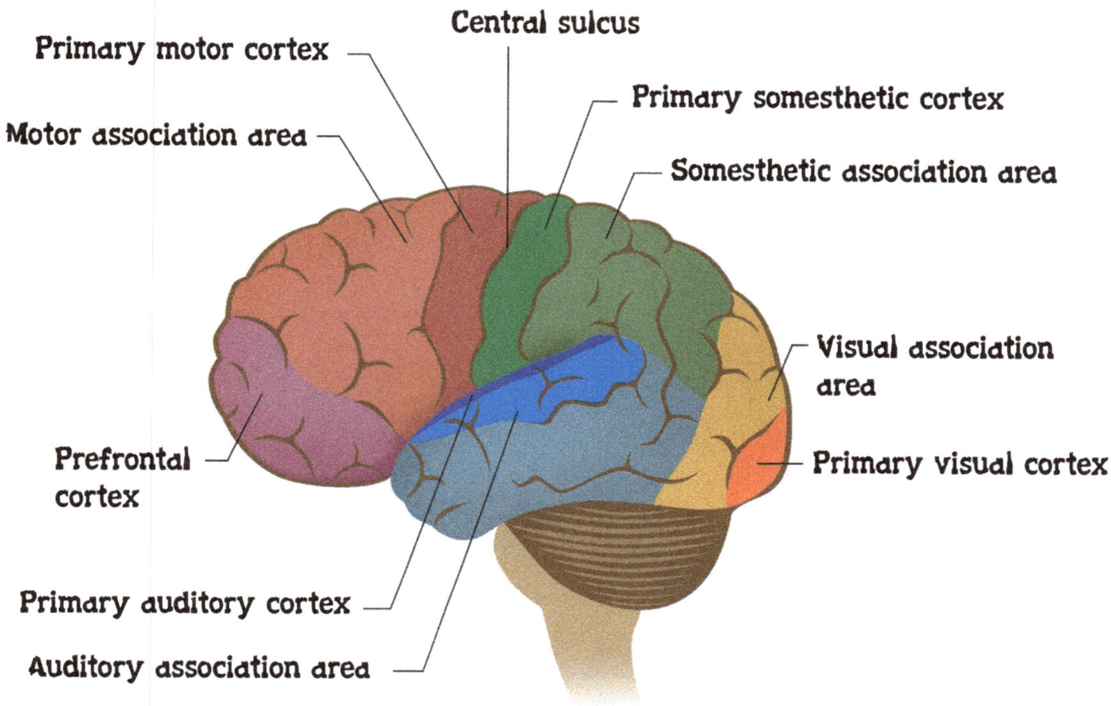

The brain works together as a whole organ, but different areas are associated with different functions. The prefrontal cortex is at the very front of the brain, behind the eyes. Once damaged by a lobotomy, the changes to the brain are permanent.

Today, surgery can be performed to treat some mental illnesses, but it is much less extreme than a lobotomy. Modern doctors may treat the most severe cases of epilepsy by cutting the corpus callosum, the structure that connects the two hemispheres of the brain. They may also treat serious depression and other mental illnesses with implants, called deep brain stimulation. These treatments can make life much better for patients, but they are only used in the most extreme cases.

The Curious Case of Phineas Gage

One of the most famous names in modern psychology and neuroscience is Phineas Gage.

In 1848, an unplanned explosion sent a tamping iron, a 13-pound (6-kilogram) metal rod, through the head of a twenty-five-year-old rail worker named Phineas Gage. The rod entered through his left eye, shot through his brain, and exited out the back of his head. Amazingly, not only did Gage survive, but witnesses reported that he didn't even lose consciousness.

It wasn't just the fact that he lived that made Phineas famous. Dr. John Martyn Harlow, who treated him after the accident, reported something truly strange had happened: Phineas's personality had changed.

Before the accident, Phineas was described as polite, soft-spoken, and responsible. After, he was short-tempered, rude, and forgetful. For the first time in modern medicine, there was evidence that a person's thoughts, feelings, and behaviors not only came from the brain, but also that injury to the brain could change a person's character.[1]

Truly Shocking!

Throughout the twentieth century, some truly shocking treatments were used for mental illness. Called "shock therapies," they used drugs and electricity to cause seizures and comas in patients and were mainly used to treat schizophrenia.

Insulin shock therapy used large injections of the hormone insulin to cause daily seizures and comas, and metrozol therapy used the drug metrozol for the same effects. These treatments were dangerous and patients suffered terrible side effects, including confusion, sweating, nausea, and dizziness.[2]

Fortunately, these treatments were used for only a couple of decades. And while they were terrible, like many medical

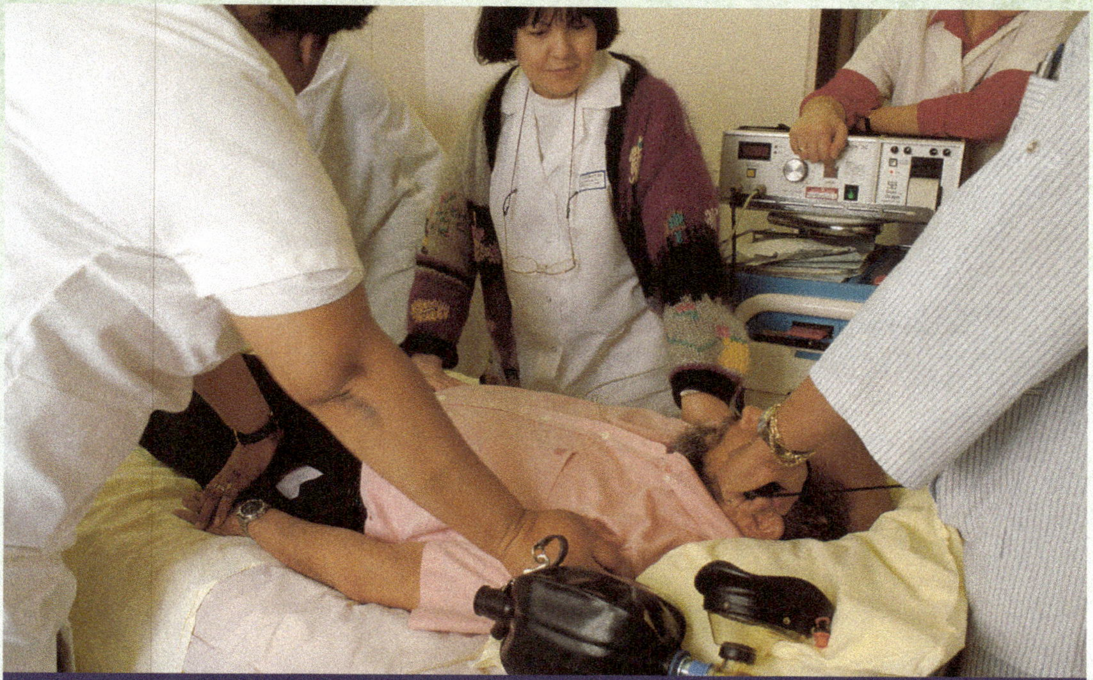

Modern electroconvulsive therapy is helpful for some patients with mental illnesses such as depression or bipolar disorder. It is done with great care so the patient is comfortable and safe. Patients are given medicine that keeps them calm and prevents them from feeling pain.

missteps, they helped lead to a much more helpful modern treatment: ECT, or electroconvulsive therapy.

Modern doctors understand that the brain is an organ, like the heart, liver, and kidneys. Just like the other organs, diseases and disorders of the brain can often be treated with medicine and healthy behavior. The brain benefits from exercise, a healthy diet, good hygiene, and modern science-based medicine just like the rest of the body.

Sadly, there is still a lot of misunderstanding around mental illness, but it is as real as illness in any other part of the body. The best ways to improve treatment of mental illness is to try to understand it.

CHAPTER 5

Bacteria: The Good, the Bad, and the Ugly

It is well known today that bacteria can cause illness. Antibacterial soaps and ointments are found in most people's medical cabinets. Antibiotics are prescribed to treat many different infections and have saved many lives. People work hard to keep things clean and sterile to prevent the spread of germs. But experts have discovered that these microorganisms can actually be helpful, and even necessary, for human health!

Bacterial Breakthrough

Bacteria are microorganisms so tiny they can be seen only with a microscope. And bacteria are everywhere. They are in the ground, in the air, in the water, in plants, and in animals. In fact, bacteria outnumber humans—even inside humans' own bodies!

All people are completely covered in and full of bacteria. If all the cells in a human body were counted, only one in ten would be human; the rest are bacteria. About 2 to 6 pounds (1 to 3 kg) of a person's bodyweight is actually made up of these creatures.

Bacteria aren't all bad. Most of the bacteria living on and inside people's bodies are good. These good bacteria work with bodies to keep them functioning and healthy.

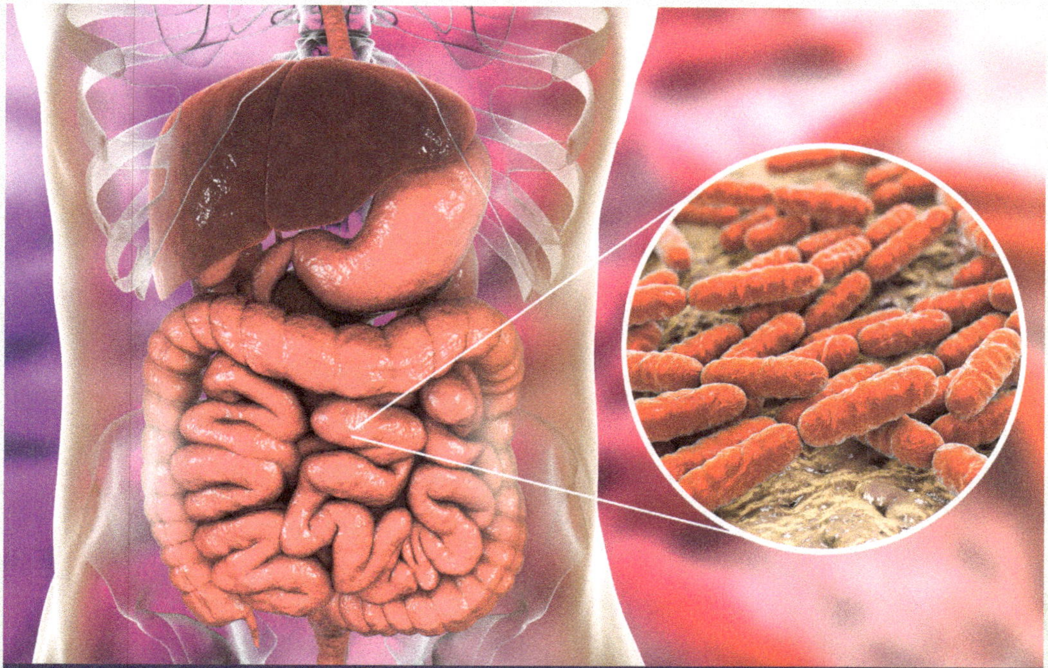

The gut, or intestines, are below the stomach and responsible for digesting food. The gut is full of bacteria. The unique ecosystem of a person's gut may affect everything from their weight to their moods!

Viral Ventures

Viruses cause many diseases, such as the common cold, the flu, and AIDS. But like bacteria, viruses have proven to be useful, too!

Retroviruses invade cells. Once inside a cell, a retrovirus changes the cell's genes. It does this by inserting a copy of its genome, or genetic makeup, into the cell's genome. Once the cells have a retrovirus in their genes, they make more of the virus every time they reproduce. This leads to infection. Scientists came up with a clever way to use the retrovirus in gene therapy. They use the retrovirus to insert medicine right into the genes of a patient's cell.

The word "bacterio-phage" means "bacteria eater." Bacteriophages are viruses that attack bacteria. Since these viruses kill bacteria but not people, they can be used to treat dangerous bacterial infections.

One of the most important jobs for bacteria in the human body is digestion. The bacteria in the gut help break down food so that the body can take in the nutrients. There are thousands of different kinds of bacteria in the gut. They make up their own biome! It's a dark, stinky, swampy ecosystem that is unique to each person. It is important to have a balance of different kinds of bacteria in the gut. Like an ecosystem in nature, the gut biome can be healthy or unhealthy, depending on the balance of bacteria.

The Poop Pill

In the past, people put poop on themselves as medicine, and that sounds preposterous. But in a case of truth being stranger than fiction, modern doctors have discovered anew the medical

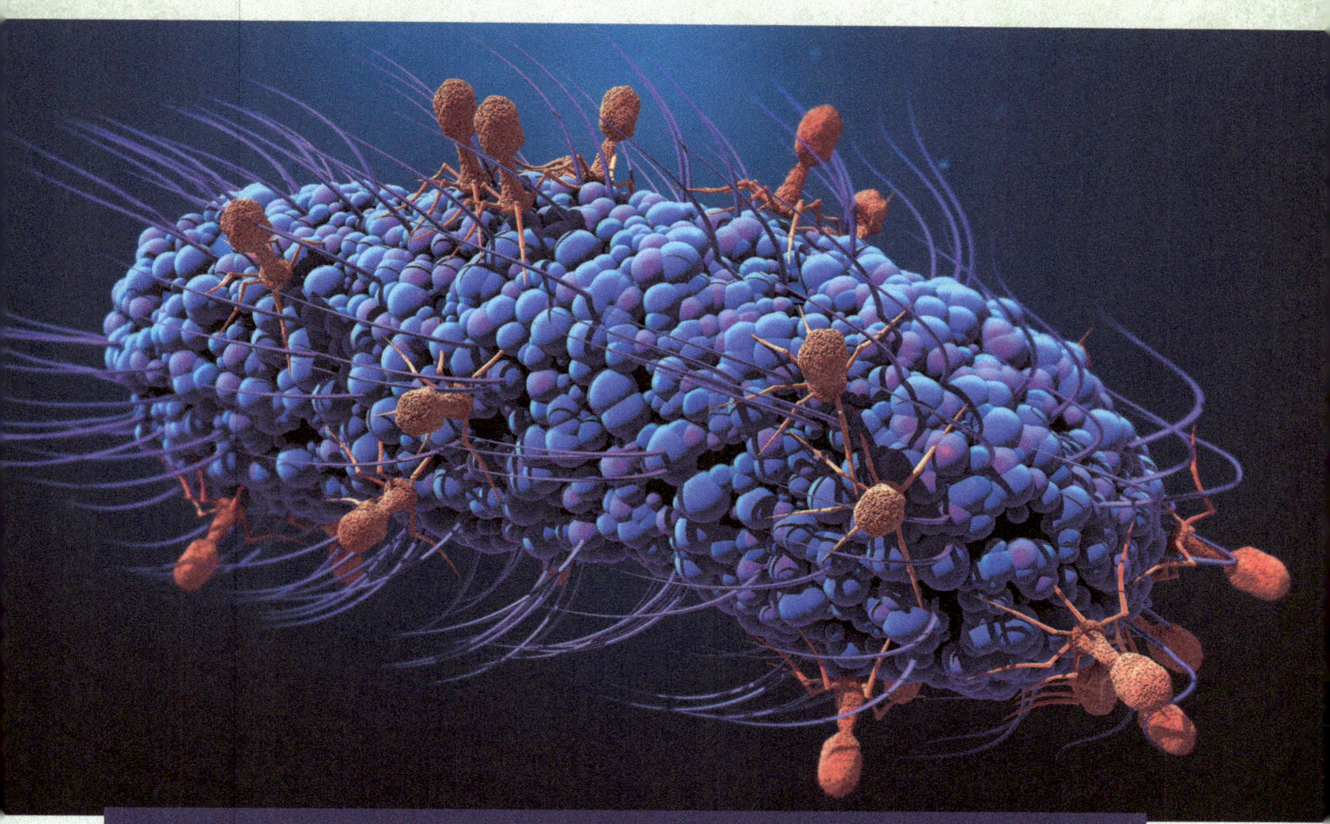

Bacteriophages, shown in red, attack a bacterium. The virions, or individual virus particles, have bulging heads that contain their DNA. Their long tails end in "tail fibers" that look a bit like spider legs.

power of poo. Feces contains gut bacteria, and doctors realized that the feces of a healthy person could be used to treat the guts of unhealthy people.

In a fecal transplant, poop from a healthy donor is frozen and made into a pill. A patient, whose gut bacteria have been damaged or destroyed, can swallow the pill to regrow their gut flora.[1] Fecal transplants are still experimental. Scientists are hopeful that they can help patients suffering from many health problems, including obesity, digestive problems such as irritable bowel syndrome (IBS), and even some neurological problems such as Parkinson's disease and multiple sclerosis (MS).

Gut Feelings

It might sound strange that a fecal transplant could help with diseases such as multiple sclerosis and Parkinson's, which affect the brain and nerves. But the gut biome affects the whole body. Scientists are still learning about all the different things it does and the way it works.

One discovery is that the gut biome communicates with the brain in unexpected ways. Scientists have discovered that the same chemicals that exist in a human brain, and are linked to thoughts and feelings, also exist in the gut. Those "gut feelings" people have are real. Some have gone so far as to call the gut the "second brain."[2] This discovery could lead down a whole new path of medicines and treatments for neurological and mental health problems!

As harmful as bad bacteria can be, they are also vital. Bacteria can even be used in making medicine. The bacteria *E. coli*, which is famous for causing food poisoning, is actually used to make life-saving insulin.[3] Insulin is a hormone that allows the energy from food to enter cells. Without insulin, people die.

People with a disease called type 1 diabetes can't make their own insulin, and they need to take insulin shots or use an insulin pump every day to stay alive. When insulin was first discovered, it was taken from pigs and cows. Animal insulin could sometimes cause allergies, and it wasn't always easy to use.

In the 1970s, scientists learned to program *E. coli* bacteria so that it would make human insulin. This is a form of genetic engineering (GM) technology. The human insulin produced by bacteria keeps millions of type 1 diabetics alive today.

Chapter Notes

Introduction

1. Tim Gower, "A Drastic Cure," *Proto*, October 3, 2015, http://protomag.com/articles/a-hole-in-the-head.

Chapter 1. Horrible History

1. Karen Carr, "The History of Indian Medicine," Quatr.us, July 22, 2017, https://quatr.us/india/history-indian-medicine.htm.
2. Mark Crislip, "Hicky: On Cupping," Science Based Medicine, April 4, 2014, https://sciencebasedmedicine.org/hickey/.
3. Rahila Bano, "Call for Hijama Therapy Regulation," BBC News, May 12, 2015, https://www.bbc.com/news/health-32653971.

Chapter 2. Gross Elixirs and Ointments

1. Dr. Joe Schwarcz, "Antimony: A Metallic Cleanse of the Middle Ages," McGill Office of Science and Society, February 15, 2017, https://www.mcgill.ca/oss/article/antimony-metallic-cleanse-middle-ages.

2. Warren R. Dawson, "Mummy as a Drug," *Proceedings of the Royal Society of Medicine*, November 21, 1927, https://www.ncbi.nlm.nih.gov/pmc/articles/PMC2101801/.
3. Orac, "Integrating Homeopathy with Medicine: Not the 'Best of Both Worlds,'" Respectful Insolence, https://respectfulinsolence.com/2018/04/20/integrating-homeopathy-with-medicine-not-the-best-of-both-worlds/.

Chapter 3. Leeches, Maggots, and Beneficial Beasts

1. Associated Press, "FDA Approves Leeches as Medical Devices," NBC News, June 28, 2004, http://www.nbcnews.com/id/5319129/ns/health-health_care/t/fda-approves-leeches-medical-devices/#.XHQIgdMrLJ8.
2. Frank Jordans, "There Are Only Two Northern White Rhinos Left. Scientists Hope Hybrid Embryos Will Save the Species," *Chicago Tribune*, July 4, 2018, https://www.chicagotribune.com/news/nationworld/science/ct-northern-white-rhino-embryos-20180704-story.html.

Chapter 4. Barbary and Bedlam

1. Steve Twomey, "Phineas Gage: Neuroscience's Most Famous Patient," *Smithsonian*, January 2010, https://www.smithsonianmag.com/history/phineas-gage-neurosciences-most-famous-patient-11390067/.

2. Madeline R. Vann, "The 10 Worst Mental Health Treatments in History," Everyday Health, March 3, 2019, https://www.everydayhealth.com/pictures/worst-mental-health-treatments-history/.

Chapter 5. Bacteria: The Good, the Bad, and the Ugly

1. Richard Klasco, "What Is a Fecal Transplant, and Why Would I Want One?" *New York Times*, January 18, 2019, https://www.nytimes.com/2019/01/18/well/live/what-is-a-fecal-transplant-and-why-would-i-want-one.html.
2. Adam Hadhazy, "Think Twice: How the Gut's 'Second Brain' Influences Mood and Well-Being," *Scientific American*, February 12, 2010, https://www.scientificamerican.com/article/gut-second-brain/.
3. Erika Gebel, "Making Insulin," Diabetes Forecast, July 2013, http://www.diabetesforecast.org/2013/jul/making-insulin.html.

Glossary

antibacterial A substance or drug that kills bacteria or prevents bacteria from growing.

bile A thick yellow or green fluid that aids in digestion.

contagious Able to spread from one person to another.

dilute To weaken by mixing with another substance, such as water.

elixir A sweetened medicinal liquid.

exorcism A practice of removing spirits or demons that are believed to possess a person or place.

flora All bacterial life in an area.

gene A unit of DNA that contains information about the traits of an organism.

genome The complete DNA of an organism.

insulin A hormone people need to turn the food they eat into energy.

microorganism A simple life form that is too small to be seen with the naked eye.

neurological Having to do with the brain and nervous system.

neuron A brain cell.

plague A disease that is highly contagious and usually fatal.

salve A healing or soothing cream.

shaman A spiritual leader and healer.

sterile Free of microorganisms.

Further Reading

Books

Cummings, Judy. *Epidemics and Pandemics: Real Tales of Deadly Diseases*. North Mankato, MN: Nomad Press, 2018.

Farndon, John. *Strange Medicine: A History of Medical Remedies*. New York, NY: Hungry Tomato, 2017.

Torres, John A. *Petrifying Plagues*. New York, NY: Enslow Publishing, 2020.

Vigliani, Marguerite, Gale Eaton, and Phillip M. Hoose. *A Story of Medicine in 50 Discoveries*. Thomaston, MN: Tilbury House Publishers, 2019.

Websites

Kidhealth

kidshealth.org/

Learn about the body, health, and medicine.

Kids.Net.Au

encyclopedia.kids.net.au/page/hi/History_of_medicine

Read more about the important people throughout the history of medicine.

***Time* for Kids**

www.timeforkids.com/g56/sections/health-and-fitness/

Explore articles about modern health, medicine, and disease outbreaks.

Index